A Poetic View of Hospice

By Marc Lerner

Introduction

In March, 2014, I had my 33rd anniversary of my diagnosis of multiple sclerosis (MS). In my 33rd year, after dealing with partial blindness, brain surgery, coping with a wheelchair and excruciating pain, I entered Hospice. My entry was not because I was expected to die soon; it was just that I was on a downhill progression with my illness and I needed to manage my pain.

It was a shock to me to be put into Hospice and I knew I had to deal with it myself. My wife, Amy, and my mom were incredible supports, but they were not always available. I used poetry as a way of coping. When issues came up, writing poetry allowed me to view that same situation from a poetic perspective.

In 2013, I wrote <u>The End: A Creative Approach to Death.</u> I felt creativity was important, because it allowed me to use my whole brain, instead of just linear thinking. I would encourage everybody to approach any major struggle using their whole brain, especially at the end of their life. It does not really matter what your creativity is, but it has to be an expression that goes beyond worry, fear or negativity.

I am not a professional poet, but I wrote these poems to help me process the dramatic journey I was on. This is the way I coped with a situation that even the experts do not have a cure for. The spiritual perspective for me was the deepest way to capture my situation not as a victim, but making the best out of a devastating situation. For those who related to my poetry, it triggered beautiful communications.

Everyone has the opportunity to utilize their right brain, if they express their heart to those they love. Only utilizing the left brain is a way to trigger frustration and a disconnect with those you love or those who love you. It is not time to focus on intellectually figuring out your situation; that needed to have been done before your final days. Completing unfinished business in your relationships is the best thing you can leave those who love you.

The following poems are an expression of the 3 months of my time in Hospice; July, 2014 to October, 2014. I am now in palliative care. My decline is not as dramatic and pain is relatively under control.

Hospice #1

My Heart Talking

Poetry was a way I regained my orientation,

For it is a way my heart talks to me

And I enter my reality with a loving connection.

There are many things that come from my heart,

But when they are in harmony with my aspirations

They stick with me independent of memory.

I can forget people places and things in my mind,

But in harmony with surrender they don't belong to me

They are gifts that come from beyond me.

Hospice #2

Surrendering

When I pass away I don't enter my idea of death,

I enter a silence that exists beyond thinking

So why is understanding what happens so important?

Understanding may help you to surrender,

But when you get there

You just let go of your mind-made reality.

Understanding may give you security,

But our real security comes from surrendering

And that is why it is the last thing you do.

Hospice #3

Best Preparation

Before I was invited into Hospice,

I prayed to God to take my life

And though I meant it Hospice took me to a different level.

Hospice turned my intentions into a reality,

Where my next step seemingly was my last

And though my body seems ready to take it I had to prepare.

Surrender is my preparation,

But standing on that threshold

Took my surrender to a deeper consciousness.

From that state of mind,

Surrender seems to touch God

And as I surrender even more… ego seems to leave.

My breath doesn't land on thoughts of "me",

It floats beyond my thoughts into silence

And the word floats indicates an effortless journey.

Keeping that experience alive for me,

Breathes life into me as I embrace it

And my exhale seems to be closer to my last.

Of course this is only symbolic,

But every thought is and we believe it

I guess this is practicing for my final journey.

Hospice #4

My Diving Board

I always say that I am ready,

But when I think of Amy

I hesitate and remember her tears.

She notes my suffering and says I can pass,

But her tears say she holds me in her heart

I am so grateful for that and I feel I'm too far to stop.

Our times together are priceless to me,

For a simple embrace takes me deep

And I realize she is the last letting go I have.

If dying was like diving off a diving board,

She is that board

So I enter the water with heartfelt love.

Hospice #5

A Preview of Passing

I woke up this morning with little memory,

I didn't know what day it was or what I was doing

I made some calls and got partially oriented but I was scared.

Was this a coming attraction of what's to come?

That is how my other handicaps were

So the only thing I could do is attempt to surrender.

That became a habit that I learned to rely on,

And if I surrender beyond my forgotten thinking

I deal with that trauma from a loving perspective.

It felt like my thinking was unplugged when my memory went,

But in a short time I remembered Amy

For she was stored in my heart.

Then I remembered Eeta, for she helps me with my work,

I am incredibly grateful

For she helps me with the work I love.

What would happen if that was permanent?

I would have a hard time dealing with my world

But I think I would feel comfortable in a loving surrender.

Maybe this is a preview of passing,

For at that time all I would want to have is surrender

Which is my highest priority and I don't think I will be there to experience it.

Hospice #6

Dealing with Pain

In illness my most profound lesson was dealing with pain,

For it forced me very deep

And I prayed Dear God please take my life.

After a month my prayers were very sincere,

But after one prayer I heard "I already did"

And it surprised me for it was not my thoughts.

It took me a while to really grasp what it meant,

For it changed the way I approached death

And instead of holding on... I let go.

If this life belongs to God,

It was easier to surrender with love

But if it was my life it was easy to hold on.

I worked on surrendering with love for decades,

But when death was not in my control

Surrender escorts me beautifully.

Hospice #7

Planning

Entering Hospice made me feel near-sighted,

For planning the future seemed so far away

And this brings me close to the moment.

In the moment I love Amy,

In fact all my love exists there

So I can't understand thoughts that take me away.

Sometimes we look forward to loving times,

But hospice turned me to seek love in the moment

So that is how I prepare for death.

I think we all need to prepare for death,

Because then we see what is temporary

And we begin to appreciate the moment more.

Sincerely approaching death,

Removes ego from the center of your life

And magically turns your center into an infinite moment.

Hospice #8

Memories

I was waiting for a cab to pick me up,

I started looking at my life in the past

And felt that I couldn't relate to it today.

When I said Dear God Take my life,

I felt when I said it this life wasn't mine

In fact I wasn't even there.

That is an amazing experience,

For it brings me closer to God

And Silence replaces me.

There pain has a unique quality,

It forces me to let go

And "I" am not included in that journey

It allows me to let go of my past,

It makes me feel as though I'm in a selfless moment

And I have no attachments.

Even with Amy and my mom,

I connect to them with love,

So my mind doesn't own our connection.

Being in Hospice I think about death often,

And that selfless moment

Is a perfect waiting room to approach death.

Hospice # 9

When to Go

Death doesn't threaten me,

For I have had tough challenges in my past

And often feel it would be better than the pain I deal with.

I share incredible moments with Amy,

And that is a stronger focus than my struggle

But as I'm steadily getting worse the future scares me.

My pain is controllable at this time,

But when it compromises our relationship and love

Death becomes more attractive.

My death would hurt Amy too much,

But when I am not able to love her

I feel death would be a gift.

Hospice #10

The Logical Boat

There is something very powerful when you are ready to give it all up,

Nothing can stop you

For in that miraculous moment you don't even exist.

The sane man doesn't want to enter it,

For sanity seems to crumble under pressure

And though pressure turns coal into diamonds sanity resists.

On the path I am on,

Turning to sanity limits what I can carry

For I have to let go and become empty for this journey.

It is when I can turn my heart inside out,

I begin to understand

The boat of logic is burning and I have to dive in to survive.

For those who hold onto their logical perspectives,

They miss the beauty of the heart

As they approach death in a burning logical boat.

Hospice #11

Searching in Silence

Tonight I finally heard the messages in these poems,

I am going to die soon

And I stopped to find a still moment to digest it.

Everything seemed to get pointless as I searched to find something,

But it wasn't a thing I was searching for

It was the acceptance of what is happening.

In many ways death seems like a relief,

But that is the spiritual side speaking

And what needs to hear it is found in a silence that never answers.

In many ways I feel I am getting closer,

And when I surrender to silence

There is nothing to be said.

Amy is a significant part of my life in times like this,

Because when I fall back on these thoughts

Our love seems to cushion my fall.

She is devastated by me dying,

But her sadness allows me not to carry unnecessary loads

And my main concern is on how Amy deals with this.

Approaching death is a great time to find depth in a relationship,

For only sincerity can speak

And only a surrendered heart can listen.

Hospice #12

Learning to Unpack

I find that preparing for death is like making a reservation,

To go somewhere very special

And after the reservation you prepare for your trip.

Instead of packing for this trip,

Because it is so special and unique

You learn how to unpack.

Preparing to die is not actually dying,

So don't file your ideas in your old folders

It is a journey we take as we surrender and wait.

For dying is not something we do,

It is given to you and all you have to do

Is receive it with a heart full of love.

Preparing to die brings you into the moment,

Where your surrender lands on love without limitations

And you can enter the Unknown with love leading the way.

This is called really resting in peace,

So after you prepare, enjoy life

Without limitations up until your last breath.

As I unpack and let go,

Surrender comes naturally.

And it feels like this is going to be a great journey.

Hospice #13

ONLY BY SURRENDER

Inner Wisdom is not at the end of linear thinking,

You get there only when you surrender

And you use your mind instead of your mind using you.

Since wisdom seldom forces its way,

You have to be incredibly sensitive to the projection of your thinking

For if it doesn't lead to the Unknown...let go of those thoughts.

When it does lead to the Unknown,

Surrendering shoehorns you perfectly into dying

And you dissolve into nothingness.

Death is your consciousness merging with the Ultimate consciousness.

Hospice #14

FOREVER

Time seems to be changing for me,

Minutes seem to be so long

And even 10 seconds seem to last forever.

Maybe that is it,

I must be getting closer to forever.

Hospice #15 Beauty Preparing for Death

I am alive feeling a beautiful connection to life,

But at the same time

The quality of the moment is compromised by my health.

My focus goes from frustration of dealing with incurable conditions with MS,

To the opposite side of the spectrum

Where I love Amy and just being with her is cause for celebration.

Now when thoughts of approaching death arise within me,

I'm going in opposite directions at the same time

And then stillness captures me.

With future problems looming over me,

My future looks not so promising

But as the negative powers increase our love does also.

As I imagine approaching death with this struggle,

It doesn't really feel as if it is my choice

So all I could do is surrender.

I know I am not quite ready yet,

Because listening instantly creates a response

But true readiness is only focused on surrendering.

No logic or excuses,

And no mourning just surrender.

Hospice #16

WILLINGNESS TO GO

When two people want to start a relationship,

They have to be willing to interact,

And that willingness allows them to go forward.

When our energies do not go toward our goal,

We naturally hold back

Which creates a resistance.

When we face death,

We have to be willing to go forward

And have our ultimate relationship.

When we are not willing,

The resistance creates anxiety

Which destroys the quality of a conscious death.

Hospice #17

THE NEGATIVE PERSPECTIVE

I once heard a person talk negatively about dying,

And all I could say is that we only love and hate ourselves

And then we share that.

The thoughts of dying exist within our brain,

So if you direct love or hate to those thoughts

You are literally loving or hating yourself.

The conscious way to approach death,

Is to develop a loving inner environment

Where entering the Unknown activates love and the end is really the end.

Hospice #18

Attempting to Fit into Dying

Thinking is like the clothes you wear,

So when you have no thoughts to focus on

You are naked.

Now nudity can be very embarrassing,

But to be embarrassed you have to focus on thinking

And when you do…you are not naked any more.

Most people never stop thinking,

But there is a real problem if you are dressed always

You can never go beyond thoughts and surrender in the moment.

Whatever you think about may be important or not,

But like our clothes they cover you

Making how you fit into society. Your priority

What if you want to fit into the Truth?

And all you can think about is your covering

That happens to most people when they think about death.

If you go beyond thinking and surrender in Silence,

You become vulnerable

Making you humble and welcomed into the Unknown.

Approaching death like this,

Makes death a comfortable next step

And in a funny way it makes being alive more complete.

Hospice #19   Dear God Take My Life

Suicide happens when you want to end your life,

It is an expression of ego or of wisdom

And when there is no surrender it is definitely ego.

One's deepest wisdom doesn't walk down that path,

It follows an invisible/thoughtless guide

Which embraces life in the moment and can do anything.

In a time of unbearable pain I prayed Dear God Please take my life,

That prayer forced me to let go of thoughts of "me",

Which really humbled me.

As time went on and my prayer persisted,

I began to really offer my life in a sincere way

And I let go of the illusion I called MY life.

To the ego that prayer is intellectual suicide,

But when you surrender

You are left in a thoughtless silence which is a rare gift.

There is what I call a conscious suicide,

An expression of inner wisdom

Where you actually find life instead of losing it.

Hospice #20

Dear God Take my Life #2

I have been asking in a prayer for God to take my life,

Sometimes immediately followed by "not in suicide"

But it had that seriousness with the intent of surrendering.

It was a prayer where consciousness leaves the thoughts I cherish,

Not the superficial ones but the ones close to my heart

And returns that consciousness that gives them life back to God.

When I am blessed to live in that reality,

I approach God loving with my whole heart

And cherish where consciousness connects me to God directly without understanding.

Dear God,

Thank You.

Hospice # 21

A Benefit of Pain

Coping with pain forced me very deep to avoid its intensity,

I was motivated to that depth not by desire or love

But by pain that drives through every block.

That journey taps the basic power of survival,

And if you are surrendered on that journey,

Without resistance you find a depth you never explored.

Arriving in silence surrendered creates an amazing gift,

There is a silence that captures you

And at that depth surrender is precious.

Often I talk about surrender as a main part of my life,

But this surrender was different

The welcome real surrender gives is like you are pulled in.

That welcome isn't in words or experience,

It pulls you deeper beyond your control

And at that depth there is just consciousness.

From there pain seems far away,

And my breath just floats through me

In fact surrender erased me.

I know this even though I was absent,

For as I returned back to my normal consciousness

Knowingness seemed to appear in my mind.

I guess pain is not all bad.

Hospice 22

Sharing Hospice

When I told Amy I was in Hospice,

She cried as if I destroyed our precious connection

But because she saw how I suffered she said it was good.

On my side of that statement,

I felt Amy's love was so dear to me

And her ability to approve was even a deeper statement of her love.

The best things in life happen beyond your control,

And the best way to allow it to happen

Is not to only focus on thinking but to follow your heart.

That doesn't mean you do nothing,

It just means the thoughts and actions you have

Comes from a surrendered place within you.

I only tell the people I trust,

For when I share what is happening

I meet them in my heart and they are genuine.

Hospice is not easy to accept,

But if approached poetically

I strengthen my commitment to live a quality life.

Hospice #23   The False Benefit of Suppression

Up until recently my need of more care has been suppressed,

Mostly by me

Because demanding it seemed to acknowledge defeat.

But when it was seen by my doctor that changed,

He saw what I needed

And that made me reluctantly accept it also.

After that acceptance,

Difficulties emerge

More than I thought and I was glad and scared.

Hospice was definitely needed,

Suppressing it had a purpose

But it wasn't good for the quality of my life.

Surrender erases personal preferences,

It takes the "you" that manipulates out

So your inner wisdom takes over.

This confronts the ego,

But that doesn't control quality

Surrender does.

Hospice #24 Real Freedom

When death is an idea,

Illusions become your coffin

And to rest in peace you have to step out of it.

A conscious death embraces silence,

For you don't hold onto any illusions.

You are totally free.

Writing poems about dying comes from my heart,

And when those ideas approach a serious reality

It is as though I lean on silence.

When you lean on your mind,

There are layers of theory backing you up

But with silence only the infinite backs you up.

You don't have to wait until you die,

To experience a conscious death

You can let go of illusions and fall into silence.

That is death to your ego,

Which is real freedom in the moment?

And that can happen many times before you die

Hospice #25 Magnetic Pull

Tonight started a new step for me,

I looked at the things I normally do

And I dropped out of those that didn't attract me.

My interest has definitely changed,

For that which involved investing time and effort

Didn't attract me at all.

In the past my work opportunities had a magnetic pull,

But that pull had no power

For my response was like talking into a dead telephone.

Creativity attracts me now with poetry and expressing my heart,

For that isn't something I do

It gets pulled out of me without effort.

When I surrender it allows the pull to be stronger,

As it feels like my heart speaking

Instead of my mind working.

That sounds like retirement,

And I feel that magnetic pull to it

But I really have to trust my heart to allow it to happen.

Hospice #26 Loving Memories

How I plan my future,

Depends on how I lived my past

But what happens when your past has little significance?

I feel my past follows me like my shadow,

It doesn't reach far back

For a shadow is just a reflection of the moment.

Of course family memories still live within me,

But what happened is harder to remember

And the value of love exists but that is a memory.

Memories of Amy are alive also,

And the memory can be found but with effort

But the experience of love covers them up.

If memories were a wall behind me,

I lean on that wall with no depth

And feel love in the moment escorts me till I die.

Memories are important,

But they are mental baggage.

And feel like obstacles as I slip into the other side.

Hospice #27

The Will to Live

When the will to love and live comes together,

And share the same breath

That moment is life's perfection.

When the will to love overshadows the will to live,

The heart is in control

But with my body it runs on flat tires and slows down.

That is the way I feel these days,

As Amy's love seems to breathe me

It is hard to climb to our normal heights.

I don't feel either of us is at fault,

My focus is just loaded

With a mixture of purposes that can't exist together.

Amy and my love is my heart's purpose,

While escaping pain is my body's

So I go in two directions in one breath.

It is like balancing on a fence between heaven and hell,

With no way to consciously choose

So I say I am ready with a heart full of love.

Hospice #28

The Purpose of Dying

The fear of death comes from the inability to control,

For "you" is not there

And the ego freaks out.

Without "you,"

There is no past history or intellect to rely on

No family or lovers and no possessions.

If there is,

You surrender to your mind

Which misses the most important surrender possible.

There is never a partial surrender,

For the part not surrendered

Is the "you" in control.

I think if you are going to die,

You have to give it your all

Otherwise it is not worth dying.

Hospice # 29

What Continues

I think our hearts are the luggage we die with,

For your love is not created by your mind

It is a pure expression of life.

Simple love is not ego's possession

It is what escorts your path in dying.

And when it is pure there are no obstacles.

So surrendering to real love,

Removes fear and resistance

So death becomes your last dance.

We dance with everything in life,

Some loving and others wild with no intimacy

If surrendered the last dance dissolves you into your partner.

If you are ready to die,

You may think "Can I have this dance?

But before you can ask you are dissolved.

Hospice # 30

Freeing Yourself from Habitual Thinking

The best thing we can do when approaching death,

Is to let go of habitual thoughts

For that frees us and makes us more conscious.

It might sound strange,

But it takes consciousness to die peacefully

For without inspiration passing is difficult.

It may sound like preparing for the future,

But that brings you into the moment

And that is where you appreciate life the most.

Even habits of prayer cannot be habitual,

For habits lack consciousness and surrender

So basically your words don't have a connection.

Our prayers are to an Ultimate consciousness,

And without connecting

God may hear us but we don't hear God.

What we don't hear may not be verbal,

But when you are receptive

Understanding may come from the inside out.

Hospice #31

Surrender as a Threshold

As I approach death,

Surrender teaches incredible lessons

And it feels like I touch what's to come.

I thought surrender was something I did,

But in a real surrender "I" doesn't exist

Which feels like a preview of death.

There are no boundaries in surrender,

For boundaries are what captures "you"

And you don't exist there.

It is impossible to imagine death,

But real surrender has no imagination

So to be empty is a threshold to dying.

Hospice #32

Surrender Determines Your Perception

When you see a picture of someone you love,

Do you surrender to what you see

Or to inner wisdom?

Perceptions are subject to your interpretations,

So ego may see something

Where wisdom sees what is there without interpretation.

True love comes without interpretations,

Which is also true for Hospice

For the ego doesn't really see what is.

Its focus comes from a mind-made reality,

Where illusions can change your perception

While inner wisdom comes from a deep inner experience.

Do I surrender to what is perceived

Or to the wisdom that perceives it?

Hospice #33

Floating Into the Future

When your future looks bleak,

You tense up as you enter

And your breath becomes choppy.

When you look out from inner wisdom,

To the same future

Your breath floats through with ease.

In Hospice when you look to the future,

When you ride that flow

The moment seems bigger as the future gets distant.

It may not be easy to walk that path,

But that tense breath isn't easy either

We just have to float into the future.

Hospice # 34

Graffiti on My Inside Walls

I have prayed for a long time to God,

Please take my life

And I heard by surprise "I already did."

Those prayers were like graffiti within me,

With sometimes desperation

And other times with frustration.

But my deepest prayers didn't have words,

It was like a silent touch

That felt like it was received.

I felt that touch when embracing Amy,

For she completely received me

And it was our love that kept me hanging on.

If illusions could save a life today,

People wouldn't die,

For that is the foundation of most people's life.

If death was a five second flash,

And we could surrender there

We could experience reality with love instead of fear.

Check your watch,

5-4-3-2-1

Enjoy.

Hospice # 35

A Final Dance

My prayers have become a subconscious habit,

I say them with pain and frustration

They automatically appear and I'm serious.

As my health gets worse and my love for Amy increases,

I seem to straddle a fence between them

While my Hospice nurse said I was in a decline.

I feel my prayer is coming sooner,

For when I close my eyes

I sense an empty space.

That tests my sincerity,

On a path you cannot turn around

And it seems to get more real.

I feel I am ready to embrace that silence,

But my heart is in Amy's hand

So I have to surrender and follow God's lead.

This final dance demands surrender,

On a very deep level

It is actually a precious gift.

For if Amy was not here feeling that,

Surrender would be sloppy

And I feel you need an accurate surrender to die.

Hospice # 36

Amy's Strength

As Amy and I digest this situation,

We cry as though our hearts are being pulled out

And because there is little to do we meet in the moment.

After a heartbroken night,

I saw her strength emerge

Without words she said I am here.

I saw her strength, in her tears,

And felt the sadness beyond them

That moment would be an amazing tool in hard times.

For just connecting to it,

We would be safe

And deal with the bigger struggles ahead of us.

Her mourning is a compliment to me,

For her heart speaks calling me with pure love

And the best I can do is being in that moment receiving it.

This drama prepares me for death,

Because we share the love that connects me to God

Making her a perfect springboard in passing.

I know Amy will struggle

I just pray she will remember her strength in that moment

For that is the part of her I cherish.

Hospice #37

A Conscious Suicide

I will consider my life over,

When I cannot love Amy with my whole heart

That will be when pain and mental confusion take over.

I would just be a burden to those who love me,

MS doesn't kill you it just makes you suffer

And that would be a worthy time to take my life.

I don't fear death like so many,

So treat me with respect

And don't project your fear onto me.

Death is a spiritual journey,

When you surrender with love connected to God

And with the pain I endure I look forward to it.

Surrendering allows me to wait until Grace moves me,

So if God is in control I can be moved to a conscious suicide

And if your God wants you to suffer you may misunderstand purpose.

Surrender connects you to God,

Which is more important than understanding

So check your connection and surrender.

Hospice #38   Sharing the Moment

When I entered the moment alone something was missing.

Understanding can't take me there

Because thoughts fall very short approaching infinity.

When going there relying on illusions,

It is like going to sleep with your lover

Wearing the clothes you wear to work.

Thinking is the clothes we cover ourselves with,

Vulnerability unlocks any door

And love is what opens the door to the moment.

When two people share the same moment,

They find a bond thoughts can never touch

And they fall into an infinite depth without being there.

Fears and doubts are like rain on the roof,

And even in a thunder storm

You don't get wet.

Amy it is our love that takes us into the moment,

And sharing it with you

Is like being served life's purpose on a silver platter.

Life can dance around us,

While a simple embrace in the moment

Is all we ever need.

Hospice #39

A Hospice Timeline

We can look at time differently,

Through the perspective of a year or a moment

The reality doesn't change but your perspective does.

Look at time in approaching death,

In a year you visit the specialist and get results from tests

And release emotions by sharing it with love ones.

In 6 months you may focus on accepting the threat differently,

For it seems to be more than an idea you need to digest

And it is getting too close to turn around.

In the moment it is amazingly different,

Here the wisdom of your body processes it

And you prepare to meet death consciously.

Ideas and beliefs are too big in a moment,

But wisdom fits perfectly

And your threat begins to be an opportunity.

Moments are easily overlooked,

Even though they represent a conscious perspective

Your ego blocks you from surrendering to it.

We can have the moment's perspective at any time,

The only requirement is

You have to let go of your conditioning so "you" doesn't exist.

Hospice # 40

Family Love Vacation

During one of my darkest weeks,

My brother and sister-in-law changed me

With simple love.

Amy and I went on a one-day vacation,

Even though it was only to downtown

It was needed to free me from my mind.

Their love attracted me,

For I tried not to talk about my illness

Even though pain was still there.

It was temporarily a vacation,

Without sharing and focusing on what was wrong

It was easy to ignore my condition.

Family love exists in the moment,

So when it consumed me

The past seldom existed.

Amy does that to me often,

I see that when ignorance blends with love

It creates a silence that dissolves any problem.

Even though that is a temporary solution,

It is always available

To free you from your mind.

Thanks Denny and Cindy.

Hospice # 41

Vacation Planning

Hospice is the ultimate vacation,

Because when dealing with your inevitable future

Important issues in the past seem to float away.

The secret of vacation is found in the word,

When you vacate your mind becomes empty.

There are no reservations needed,

For it feels like it has already been planned

So all you need to do is surrender.

You don't need to pack,

For "vacate" leaves you empty

In the ultimate vacate you don't exist.

This vacation isn't in time and space,

For when there is no "you"

There is nowhere to go.

Hospice # 42

Intimate Foreplay

Making love and dying are harmonious opposites,

For one is entering and one is exiting

But they both require conscious foreplay.

Both require intimate love,

For a loving foreplay in making love

Provides conscious entry which is essential for real quality.

When facing the threat of death loving foreplay is also important

Here poetry prepares me

For that is how I will have a conscious passing.

Foreplay in making love,

Demands intimacy

For without it the act is like rape.

Foreplay in dying prepares you also,

For it eliminates useless anxiety

And turns it into a spiritual experience.

It is kind of funny,

For with conscious intimacy

You don't know if you are coming or going.

Hospice #43

An Evolved Prayer

When it was like each breath triggered pain,

My prayer was

Dear God please take my life.

That was years ago and many bouts of gratitude,

My prayer stays the same

But now life equals consciousness.

Allowing God to take your consciousness,

Is a wonderful surrender

Not of this or that but of your whole life.

For without consciousness,

You are not aware of anything

That is the way we give our life to God totally.

You are still alive,

But surrendered

Living a life with love from a depth where God is in every breath.

That is how I live with pain,

And that is a great price to pay to get there

But it is worth it.

Hospice #44

Erasing the Eraser

Sometimes I look at my life

And would like to erase my thoughts and actions

But when I surrender I want to erase the eraser.

It is not that I don't want to exist,

I just love the silence that stops ego's expressions

As life flows through and expresses itself.

A magic moment in life happens when two lives embrace,

That is an example where I do not exist

I think that happens in the simplicity of Amy's and my love.

When we connect,

It feels like a doorway that opens into infinity

As my identity dissolves into nothingness.

Hospice #45

Making Death Nauseous

Do you need someone there to feel love?

To pray without a congregation?

To care without rewards?

If you do, it is hard to die alone.

Our final state of mind,

Is empty

Which allows me to be swallowed completely.

If mind isn't empty,

Death chokes

And throws up to start again.

Hospice #46

Fear of Death

I got a glimpse at what creates the fear of death today,

When I was organizing my Birthday party

I felt the love & good feelings from friends & resisted leaving.

The reality of what surrounded me was so real,

It would be hard to replace it

With the unknown.

That would be true even if my reality wasn't good,

For replacing anything with uneasiness

Jams the mind and fear emerges.

If you looked forward to the life after death,

It may be possible to trade

So you are seemingly happy to pass.

To really be convinced the past is a step better,

Your experience cannot be theatrical

That experience has to be pure and not a creation of your mind.

*

Hospice #47

Being a Puppet

When I was in intense pain I had a prayer,

Dear God take my life

It became a habit but it was sincere.

When the pain became tolerable

The same prayer still emerged but with a deeper meaning.

I was alive and having God take my life,

Meant ego didn't limit me

And I served like a hand puppet.

When God was the hand,

My thoughts and actions didn't seem as mine

And the pain wasn't mine either.

That was a perfect preparation for death

Because I identified with what I was to merge into.

When there is no stepping stone between life and death,

There is no resistance

As surrender leads the way.

*

Hospice #48

The Beauty of a Damaged Ego

Let me try to share a benefit of a damaged ego,

It happens when you deal with a constant threat like an illness

And no matter what you do it doesn't go away.

You are stuck looking through the eyes of frustration,

Which basically captures ego's effort to improve

But when you transcend ego...you are truly blessed.

Unfortunately society runs on ego,

Which is celebrated

Rather than being defeated and ignored.

The damaged ego is easier to transcend,

For when you are sick it isn't your fault

And it is seen as your strength rather than defeat.

This is a hidden blessing in poor health,

For when your ego is strong and rewarding

Transcending it is difficult.

Everyone desires sharing pure love,

Transcending a damaged ego

Opens a path where pure love can flow.

I know people who are loving and have a healthy ego,

They can transcend it to a certain point

But this is an endless journey never complete until you die.

Hospice #49 What Does This Mean?

A phenomenon has captured my attention,

I have been writing about it for years

And when it appeared it took me by surprise.

I drifted into a state where I was conscious

But I didn't exist.

I could hear Amy talking,

But "I" had no interpretations of it

And though it looked like I was sleeping I was conscious.

The "me" which I identified with wasn't part of the picture,

Stillness seemed to fill it up as silence was the background.

Intimacy and fatigue opened the door to that moment,

And without any resistance]

The moment captured me.

Amy saw this happen several times,

She often said "come back"

And I returned to a normal state of being.

Only when she was there did I remember what happened,

Which makes me think

This could have happened when I was alone also.

It was Amy that gave me that intimacy,

And coming back to her allowed me to remember what happened

What would it be like to live like that?

What if the two states of being happened at once?

Was that a stepping stone into the future?

Hospice #50

Strengthening the Will to Live

To be loved and respected is like a touch to your heart,

It strengthens your will to live

And when it is returned it becomes mystical.

People can praise and even honor your ego,

But that is the mind talking to the mind

Which is a symbolic touch that activates the brain.

An active brain is like runners passing a baton,

Though they connect

Their focus on each other is temporary.

Both connections can strengthen the will to live,

But the will to live strengthened with the heart

Brings a quality to life that leads to a conscious passing.

From that perspective,

It isn't that you <u>want</u> to die

It's more like you live fully till it is over.

Hospice #51

Yom Kippur Prayer

As I approach one of the holy days as a Jew,

Yom Kippur

I am alone with God and feel ready...

On one level I'm ready to enter a year of connection,

In a sense of surrender

Which opens a channel from my heart to God.

On another level I am prepared to die,

Which is very similar

But it feels like an endless journey of surrender.

Opening the channel to God is sacred,

And giving yourself completely

Has to include your life unconditionally.

To me in my condition it is dying,

But dying without any conditions

Means I have no control of when I pass.

But doesn't mean God can't lead me to do anything,

And how do I know it isn't my choice?

I pray my last breath is complete,

As it rises from a deep Surrender

And that is all I can do.

Hospice #52   How I Love

I have prayed to surrender for years,

My prayer was

Dear God take my life and my heart.

I felt as though my life started to leave,

And surrender was to let go

Instead of holding onto thoughts.

Holding onto life is celebrated,

But letting go of my life is right

As my consciousness entered God.

Amy is all I would hold onto,

But discomfort outweighed that attachment

And I let go.

Amy may not understand this poem,

But if God took my heart

It was my love for God that bonded us together.

We cherished our love together,

For loving God

Is constant and unconditional.

That is how I loved Amy,

Not consciously

But as a bi-product of loving God.

Hospice #53

An Endless Flow

Dear God please take my life,

Was a phrase that dealt with discomfort and pain

And it began as a suicidal thought but began to change.

The willingness to give my life was significant,

For it forced my ego out of my focus

And was replaced by silence.

When that happened that prayer turned spiritual,

It was like God pulled consciousness from me,

And I merged.

Without ego life is consciousness,

That is what real surrender is

And that is impossible with the fear of dying.

The willingness to give your all precedes surrender,

If not there you don't let go of life

And you automatically hold onto thinking.

Without surrender your breath bounces,

And with surrender it floats till it stops

And that is how you embrace life without trying.

The opposite of silence is thinking,

Something the inquisitive ego can't understand

But true surrender doesn't need explanation.

Life just happens,

As surrender flows with it

And all one does is casually flow within

Hospice #54 Dealing with Pain

Getting used to pain,

Is like living in a dysfunctional home with violence

And though you get used to it life is empty.

Time stops with pain,

The moment demands attention

As the past and future easily slip away.

Once you adapt to it,

There is a spiritual blessing in it

For the moment becomes where you live.

Not that the moment is rewarding physically

But you live here and now.

An empty here and now has benefits also,

When not focused on "things"

Thinking loses your focus also.

Then awareness sinks deeper within,

And instead of you grasping reality

Reality seems to grasp you.

Then surrender is all you can do,

And for that moment

You don't exist but you feel complete.

That is when I forget I'm in Hospice,

And though pain still exists

I breathe an easy breath.

Hospice # 55 Loving Interactions

When spending time alone,

I don't think of my struggle very often

But when interacting it is natural to express oneself.

How intimate you are with them,

Determines the depth you share

But even with your lover there are other considerations.

A true lover sometimes requires deep sensitivity,

For if you flirt with death and it hurts them

Knowing they are with you every step you take your heart has to talk.

Your connection to them is the most important thing,

For sensitivity to their struggle

Allows them to be selfless to the end.

This journey requires both to be conscious,

For time in hospice requires incredible strength

And ego's frustration is just selfish.

Loving interaction is your best medicine,

And when your heart speaks

You dance with grace as if it was the music.

Amy and I spent days in that space this weekend,

And though it seemed like we did nothing

Times like that are like a miracle cure that effortlessly happened.

That time was beautiful making life seemingly endless,

And though we know there is an end

Every breath was a celebration that was magical.

Hospice #56   Looking

The simple act of losing something,

While in Hospice

Is different.

It seems easier to let go of it,

Without panic

And seems natural.

The normal reaction of planning something else,

Is replaced by forgetting what happened

And you just sit and wait.

I don't know what I am waiting for,

It never is found in a blank stare

But too often that's what happens.

If I had something to do that interested me,

That stare would turn into thinking

And a normal life would continue.

I am bored with being sick,

But I do not have a choice

I just have to remember the magic exists in every moment.

That magic is not found in memory,

And looking for it doesn't help either

Simply being in the moment blesses you with that quality.

And that is where magic comes in,

And all you have to do is receive it.

Hospice #57

The Touch

To be loved and respected is like a touch to your heart,

It strengthens your will to live

And when it is returned it becomes mystical.

People can praise and even honor your ego,

But that is the mind talking to the mind

Which is a symbolic touch that activates the brain.

An active brain is like runners passing a baton,

Though they connect

Their focus on each other is temporary.

Both connections can strengthen the will to live,

But the will to live strengthened with the heart

Brings a quality to life that leads to a conscious passing.

From that perspective,

It isn't that you <u>want</u> to die

It's more like you live fully till it is over.

Hospice # 58

A Poetic View of Hospice

When your right brain embraces the Unknown,

Though you might not die right away

Creativity offers great comfort.

After three months in Hospice,

I truly benefitted

It was like looking in the mirror at my depth.

I had no plans for the future,

No regrets of the past

I was just trapped in the moment.

Instead of worrying about my health,

I occupied my time with poetry which helped me to step aside

And watched inner wisdom comfort me.

This changed the end which normally scares people,

But for me I approach death being open

Not knowing what exists I just surrender.

Hospice discharged me and I returned to palliative care,

But my health stayed the same

And this journey gave me a perspective that includes all of me.

Most people do not have the opportunity to face death,

But when you do

You really appreciate your life in a tender way.

My Creative Path

In 1981, I was diagnosed with multiple sclerosis. The way I coped with my poor health was to be creative in dealing with the problems my illness gave me. Then, when the techniques I developed worked for me, I shared them with others in a struggle. I worked through a non-profit organization and dealt with three groups.

First, I worked for twenty-five years with Vietnam combat veterans who had PTSD and were my age. They related to me because both of our struggles were incurable by the experts. I learned the most from this group, because they knew how to fight for their life. When they were in combat, they were forced to a super-conscious state of mind. Unfortunately, they lost it as they re-entered society. My main approach to these veterans was to help them re-own that state of mind to deal with the struggles they faced. More veterans died from suicide after the war then were lost in the war itself. Now, they had to fight for their life in a different way.

The second group was the mentally ill homeless in Santa Monica, California. The challenge I had with this group was to make what I presented very simple. Actually, this helped me relate to everyone in a struggle, because when their struggle was intense, it affected their ability to concentrate. I liked working with this group because, when they trusted you, they became very open to learn.

The third group was people who dealt with life-threatening illnesses, like AIDS and cancer. Many in this group had developed intellects and it was difficult for them to be simple. I felt being simple and direct bypassed the layer of the mind that protected them. They had to let go of that protection and allow direct work on their body, because that is where the real work had to happen.

Working and sharing what helped me allowed me to write four books.

- <u>A Healthy Way to Be Sick</u>, where experiential exercise will direct you to work on your health. You will learn the value of silence in the healing process. The main part of healing is trusting yourself. A main technique in this book will teach you self-trust. The final technique is learning to use your mind as a Bio-computer. This is where you program the techniques you learn; awareness is the input, which connects to the program and corrections automatically happen.

- <u>The Positive Self: Change Your Self-Image and You Change Your Life</u> helps you to have the best part of you involved in your struggle. This is the part of you that relies on the Wisdom of the Body more than your past conditioning. It has clarity in thinking and understanding, which empowers you to be an active partner with your doctor. The Positive Self will develop the life skills needed to in healing.

- <u>The End, A Creative Way to Approach Death</u> is a book that was written after brain surgery and intense pain. I appreciated a creative way to live and to heal. Now I wanted to have a creative way to approach death. When I faced death directly with a creative perspective, I embraced life in a very special way.

- <u>A Poetic View of Hospice</u> is a way I coped with the idea of being in Hospice. I learned in the past that this is where people go before they die. My illness was getting worse, but it did not feel like I had six months to live. These poems untangled my mind, inspired me, and helped me focus on having a quality life until I die.

All of these books are available on Amazon/Kindle.com. Search by title or author.

www.ingramcontent.com/pod-product-compliance
Lightning Source LLC
Chambersburg PA
CBHW080324290526
45793CB00006B/1204